BOOK DESCRIPTION: 4

BOOK DESCRIPTION: 4

INTRODUCTION 6

CHAPTER 1: FUNDAMENTALS OF BODY FLUIDS 8
    1.1 BODY WATER COMPOSITION 9
    1.2 FLUID COMPARTMENTS 11
    1.3 FLUID MOVEMENT 13
    1.4 FLUID BALANCE 15

CHAPTER 2: ELECTROLYTES IN ACTION 18
    2.1 UNDERSTANDING ELECTROLYTES 19
    2.2 MAJOR ELECTROLYTES AND THEIR ROLES 21
    2.3 ELECTROLYTE HOMEOSTASIS 24
    2.4 CLINICAL IMPLICATIONS OF IMBALANCES 26
    2.5 CASE STUDIES 29

CHAPTER 3: ACID-BASE BALANCE EXPLAINED 32
    3.1 BASICS OF pH AND ITS IMPORTANCE 33
    3.2 ACID PRODUCTION AND ELIMINATION 35
    3.3 BUFFER SYSTEMS 38
    3.4 RESPIRATORY AND RENAL CONTRIBUTIONS 40
    3.5 RECOGNIZING AND CORRECTING IMBALANCES 43

CHAPTER 4: INTEGRATION OF FLUIDS, ELECTROLYTES, AND ACID-BASE BALANCE 47
    4.1 INTERCONNECTIONS AND THEIR IMPORTANCE 48
    4.2 FLUID AND ELECTROLYTE DISORDERS 50
    4.4 TREATMENT STRATEGIES 54
    4.5 SIMULATED PATIENT SCENARIOS 56

CHAPTER 5 PRACTICAL APPLICATIONS 60
    5.1 DAILY APPLICATIONS 61
    5.2 ADVANCED MONITORING TECHNIQUES 63
    5.3 THE FUTURE OF FLUID AND ELECTROLYTE MANAGEMENT 66
    5.4 CONTINUOUS LEARNING 68
    5.5 REVIEW AND SELF-ASSESSMENT 69

CONCLUSION 71

Fluids and Electrolytes

A Fast and Easy Way to Understand Acid-Base Balance without Memorization

© Copyright 2024 - All rights reserved.

The content contained within this book may not be reproduced, duplicated or transmitted without direct written permission from the author or the publisher.

Under no circumstances will any blame or legal responsibility be held against the publisher, or author, for any damages, reparation, or monetary loss due to the information contained within this book. Either directly or indirectly.

Legal Notice:

This book is copyright protected. This book is only for personal use. You cannot amend, distribute, sell, use, quote or paraphrase any part, or the content within this book, without the consent of the author or publisher.

Disclaimer Notice:

Please note the information contained within this document is for educational and entertainment purposes only. All effort has been executed to present accurate, up to date, and reliable, complete information. No warranties of any kind are declared or implied. Readers acknowledge that the author is not engaging in the rendering of legal, financial, medical or professional advice. The content within this book has been derived from various sources. Please consult a licensed professional before attempting any techniques outlined in this book.

By reading this document, the reader agrees that under no circumstances is the author responsible for any losses, direct or indirect, which are incurred as a result of the use of information contained within this document, including, but not limited to, — errors, omissions, or inaccuracies.

Book Description:

Are you struggling to grasp the complexities of fluids, electrolytes, and acid-base balance in your healthcare studies or practice? Do traditional methods of memorization leave you feeling overwhelmed and unsure when it comes to applying this knowledge in real-world situations?

"Fluids and Electrolytes: A Fast and Easy Way to Understand Acid-Base Balance without Memorization" is your solution. This book takes an innovative approach to teaching these critical concepts, focusing on practical understanding rather than rote learning.

In this book, you will:

- **Master the Basics:** Learn the foundational principles of fluid balance, electrolyte functions, and acid-base regulation through clear, straightforward explanations.

- **Apply Knowledge Clinically:** Discover how to connect theoretical knowledge to everyday clinical scenarios, enabling you to make informed decisions with confidence.

- **Visualize Complex Concepts:** Benefit from diagrams, charts, and real-world examples that make learning easier and more intuitive.

- **Skip the Memorization:** Understand the relationships between fluids, electrolytes, and acid-base balance without relying on complicated formulas or extensive memorization.

- **Improve Patient Outcomes:** Equip yourself with the tools and knowledge needed to manage these critical elements effectively in any healthcare setting, from routine care to emergency situations.

Whether you are a nursing student, a seasoned nurse, or a healthcare professional looking to refresh your knowledge, this book provides you with the essential skills to excel in your field. It's not just about passing exams; it's about mastering the material in a way that sticks and makes a real difference in patient care.

Prepare to transform your understanding and approach to fluids, electrolytes, and acid-base balance—without the stress of memorization.

Introduction

Fluids, electrolytes, and acid-base balance are the foundation of life. These elements are the driving forces behind every heartbeat, every breath, and every cellular function in the human body. Without them, the body's intricate systems would fail, leading to severe consequences. Understanding these components is not just academic; it's a matter of life and death in healthcare. Mastering the balance of fluids and electrolytes, as well as the body's pH, is crucial for anyone involved in patient care, from routine check-ups to emergency interventions.

For healthcare professionals, the ability to manage fluids, electrolytes, and acid-base balance is critical. These topics are not just theoretical—they are at the heart of clinical practice. Whether adjusting IV fluids, interpreting lab results, or responding to a patient in crisis, a deep understanding of these concepts can mean the difference between effective treatment and life-threatening errors. Nurses, doctors, and paramedics must make quick, informed decisions about a patient's fluid and electrolyte status. Misjudging a patient's hydration levels, or failing to recognize an acid-base imbalance, can lead to serious, sometimes fatal, outcomes. This knowledge is foundational in fields ranging from emergency medicine to chronic disease management, and it is a skill set that every healthcare provider must master. Understanding how these elements interact within the body allows professionals to anticipate complications, personalize care, and improve patient outcomes consistently. Whether managing dehydration in an elderly patient or correcting acidosis in the ICU, proficiency in these areas is essential for high-quality care.

Learning about fluids, electrolytes, and acid-base balance often feels daunting, even for seasoned healthcare professionals. The complexity of these topics lies in the intricate physiological mechanisms that govern the body's balance, often requiring an understanding of various systems working together. Many students and practitioners struggle with the traditional approach to learning these concepts, which often relies heavily on memorization of formulas, lab values, and processes. This method can lead to confusion and frustration, especially when attempting to apply this knowledge in real-world clinical settings.

One of the most common challenges is the overwhelming amount of detail involved. Students may find themselves bogged down by the need to remember specific electrolyte concentrations, normal ranges, and the corresponding effects of deviations. Additionally, the interconnected nature of these topics—where a change in one area can significantly impact another—can make it difficult to see the bigger picture. This can result in a fragmented understanding that doesn't translate well into practical application, leaving many feelings uncertain and unprepared when faced with real patient scenarios.

This book takes a different approach. Rather than focusing on rote memorization, it emphasizes a practical understanding of the core principles. The goal is to simplify complex concepts by breaking them down into easily digestible parts and connecting them to everyday clinical situations. Instead of memorizing formulas, you will learn to understand the relationships between fluids, electrolytes, and acid-base balance through clear explanations, visual aids, and relatable examples. This method not only makes the material more accessible but also more applicable, enabling you to make quick, accurate decisions in a clinical setting. By the end of this book, you will have the confidence to handle these challenges with ease, applying your knowledge effectively in your day-to-day practice.

Chapter 1: Fundamentals of Body Fluids

1.0 Introduction to Body Fluids

Why does a deep understanding of body fluids matter for anyone pursuing a career in healthcare? From regulating temperature to transporting nutrients and waste, the fluids circulating within our bodies play a pivotal role in nearly every physiological process. This chapter will equip you with foundational knowledge about body fluids, focusing on their composition, the different compartments they occupy, their movement throughout the body, and how they maintain balance—an essential baseline for any medical professional.

Objectives:

- Understand the basic concepts of body fluid composition and the significance of various fluid compartments.
- Learn the dynamics of fluid movement and the mechanisms behind fluid balance.
- Prepare to apply this knowledge in clinical settings to enhance patient care.

Overview: We will start by exploring the total body water, illustrating its distribution and factors affecting its composition. Then, we will define the primary fluid compartments, delving into their specific functions and the solutes they contain. Following that, we'll examine how fluids move within and between these compartments and conclude with an overview of how the body maintains fluid balance through various physiological mechanisms. This foundational knowledge sets the stage for more complex discussions in subsequent chapters and provides the tools needed to tackle clinical challenges effectively.

1.1 Body Water Composition

Total body water (TBW) is a fundamental concept in understanding human physiology, representing the sum of all fluids within a person's body. It typically accounts for about 60% of an adult's total weight, though this percentage can vary significantly across different age groups, genders, and body compositions.

Total Body Water Distribution:

- **Adult Males:** Approximately 60% of their body weight.

- **Adult Females:** Slightly lower, about 50-55%, mainly due to a higher proportion of body fat.

- **Infants:** As high as 75-78%, decreasing gradually to adult levels.

Factors Affecting Body Water Composition:

1. **Age:** Infants and young children have higher percentages of body water than adults, which decreases with age. The elderly often have reduced body water, making them more susceptible to dehydration.

2. **Gender:** Men typically have higher body water percentages than women due to having more lean muscle mass and less body fat.

3. **Body Fat:** Individuals with a higher body fat percentage typically have less body water since adipose tissue contains less water than muscle.

Visualizing Variations: To aid in understanding, consider the following table that illustrates TBW variations among different populations:

Population Group	Percentage of Body Water
Newborn Infants	75-78%
Adult Males	60%
Adult Females	50-55%
Elderly	Below 50%

This variation is crucial for healthcare providers to recognize because it affects hydration status assessments, fluid replacement therapies, and the management of various medical conditions.

In clinical practice, understanding these factors helps in accurately assessing a patient's hydration needs. For example, an elderly woman may require a more cautious approach to fluid replacement than a young adult male, due to her naturally lower body water content and potential for chronic illnesses that may complicate fluid balance.

By the end of this section, you should have a clear understanding of how total body water is distributed and the factors that influence its composition, equipping you with the knowledge to make informed decisions in managing patient care.

1.2 Fluid Compartments

The human body is primarily composed of water, which is distributed in two main fluid compartments: the intracellular fluid (ICF) and the extracellular fluid (ECF). Understanding the characteristics of these compartments is essential for any healthcare professional as they directly influence how substances are transported in the body, how cells function, and how treatments are administered.

Intracellular Fluid (ICF):

- **Definition:** ICF refers to the fluid contained within cells, making up about two-thirds of the total body water in humans.

- **Volume:** In an average adult, the ICF accounts for approximately 25 to 40 liters of fluid.

- **Function:** ICF is crucial for maintaining cell integrity and function. It acts as the medium in which cellular processes occur, including energy production, metabolism, and protein synthesis.

- **Key Solutes:** Potassium (K^+), Magnesium (Mg^{2+}), and Phosphate (HPO_4^{2-}) are predominant in the ICF. These solutes play critical roles in cell function, including maintaining electrical charge and osmotic balance, which are essential for muscle contraction, nerve impulse transmission, and cellular energy storage.

Extracellular Fluid (ECF):

- **Definition:** ECF includes all body fluids outside cells, divided into two subcategories: interstitial fluid, which surrounds and bathes the cells, and plasma, the liquid component of blood.

- **Volume:** The ECF volume is about one-third of the total body water, roughly 15 to 20 liters in an average adult.

- **Function:** ECF serves primarily as a transport medium for nutrients, waste products, and other substances between blood vessels and cells. It also plays a critical role in maintaining proper osmotic pressure and fluid balance within the body.

- **Key Solutes:** Sodium (Na+), Chloride (Cl-), and Bicarbonate (HCO3-) dominate the ECF. Sodium is particularly important for fluid balance, nerve function, and muscle function. Chloride helps maintain cellular integrity and fluid balance, while bicarbonate regulates pH.

The interaction between these compartments and their solutes facilitates vital physiological functions, such as the transmission of nerve impulses, muscle contractions, and the regulation of pH. Any imbalance in the distribution of these solutes can lead to disorders such as dehydration, edema, and acidosis or alkalosis, making the knowledge of fluid compartments foundational for diagnosing and treating these conditions effectively.

By understanding the volumes, functions, and key solutes of these compartments, healthcare professionals can better manage fluid therapy, recognize the signs of electrolyte imbalances, and ensure optimal patient outcomes.

1.3 Fluid Movement

Fluid movement within the human body is governed by several mechanisms that are essential for maintaining cellular function and overall fluid balance. These mechanisms include osmosis, diffusion, and active transport, each playing a crucial role in the distribution of fluids and solutes across cellular membranes and within different body compartments.

Osmosis:

- **Definition:** Osmosis is the movement of water across a semipermeable membrane from an area of lower solute concentration to one of higher solute concentration.

- **Contribution to Fluid Balance:** This process helps maintain the balance of water between the intracellular and extracellular compartments, crucial for cell survival and function.

- **Example:** In dehydration, the extracellular fluid becomes more concentrated with solutes due to reduced water intake. Osmosis causes water to move out of the cells to balance the solute concentrations, potentially leading to cell shrinkage and dysfunction.

Diffusion:

- **Definition:** Diffusion is the movement of solutes from an area of higher concentration to an area of lower concentration, not necessarily involving a membrane.

- **Contribution to Fluid Balance:** Diffusion allows for the equalization of solute concentrations, aiding in the transport of nutrients, gases, and waste products across cells and tissues.

- **Example:** In the lungs, oxygen diffuses from the alveoli, where it is at a higher concentration, into the blood, where its concentration is lower. This is essential for oxygen delivery to tissues.

Active Transport:

- **Definition:** Unlike osmosis and diffusion, active transport requires energy (ATP) to move solutes against their concentration gradient, through a membrane from lower to higher concentration.

- **Contribution to Fluid Balance:** Active transport is critical for maintaining essential gradients, particularly in nerve and muscle cells, and for the absorption and secretion of nutrients and ions in various organs.

- **Example:** In the kidneys, sodium ions are actively transported out of the renal tubules back into the blood, a process crucial for regulating blood volume and pressure. This transport also influences the passive reabsorption of water and other solutes, playing a key role in fluid and electrolyte balance.

These mechanisms collectively ensure that essential substances are distributed properly throughout the body, maintaining homeostasis. For instance, in patients receiving IV therapy, osmosis and diffusion dictate how fluids distribute between the bloodstream and cellular spaces, affecting hydration status and drug efficacy. Active transport mechanisms, such as those in the kidneys and digestive tract, further refine this balance by selectively retaining or excreting substances based on the body's needs. Understanding these processes is vital for devising effective treatments in clinical settings, such as adjusting fluid and electrolyte therapy in response to changes in patient status.

1.4 Fluid Balance

Fluid balance is a critical aspect of homeostasis, the body's ability to maintain internal stability despite external changes. This balance involves the precise regulation of the body's fluid volumes, solute concentration, and pressures within its fluid compartments, ensuring optimal functioning of cells and organs.

Importance of Fluid Balance: Maintaining fluid balance is essential for numerous physiological functions, including temperature regulation, transport of nutrients and waste products, and overall cellular health. Disruptions in fluid balance can lead to significant health issues, ranging from minor ailments to life-threatening conditions.

Organ Roles in Fluid Regulation:

1. **Kidneys:** The primary regulators of fluid balance, kidneys adjust the volume and composition of body fluids by filtering blood, reabsorbing necessary substances, and excreting waste and excess water in urine. They respond dynamically to changes in hydration status, ensuring that the internal environment remains stable.

2. **Skin:** Through perspiration, the skin not only helps regulate body temperature but also assists in fluid balance. Sweating results in water loss, which can be significant during intense exercise or high temperatures.

3. **Lungs:** Every breath exhales a small amount of water vapor, contributing to fluid loss. The lungs also play a role in maintaining acid-base balance, which is closely linked to fluid and electrolyte balance.

4. **Gastrointestinal Tract:** Fluid intake and absorption primarily occur in the GI tract, while fluid loss happens

through feces. Disorders that increase fluid loss via the GI tract, such as diarrhea, can rapidly upset fluid balance.

Hormonal Regulation of Fluid Balance: Several hormones are instrumental in regulating fluid and electrolyte balance:

- **Antidiuretic Hormone (ADH):** Produced by the pituitary gland, ADH signals the kidneys to increase water reabsorption when the body is dehydrated, helping to concentrate the urine and conserve water.

- **Aldosterone:** Secreted by the adrenal cortex, aldosterone prompts the kidneys to retain sodium and water, while excreting potassium, thus influencing blood volume and pressure.

- **Atrial Natriuretic Peptide (ANP):** This heart-produced hormone opposes the action of aldosterone, promoting the excretion of sodium and water, which decreases blood volume and pressure.

Common Disruptions in Fluid Balance:

- **Dehydration:** Caused by insufficient fluid intake or excessive fluid loss (through sweating, diarrhea, or vomiting), dehydration manifests with symptoms like thirst, reduced urine output, dry skin, fatigue, and dizziness. Severe dehydration can lead to kidney failure, seizures, and hypovolemic shock.

- **Fluid Overload:** Excessive fluid intake or compromised fluid excretion (due to heart, kidney, or liver disease) can lead to fluid overload. Symptoms include swelling, breathing difficulties, and altered mental status. Chronic cases can exacerbate heart failure and pulmonary edema.

Understanding these mechanisms is crucial for healthcare providers, as maintaining or restoring fluid balance is a fundamental aspect of patient care. Effective management of fluid balance can significantly improve outcomes in a wide range of clinical scenarios, from surgical recovery to chronic disease management.

Chapter 2: Electrolytes in Action

2.0 Introduction to Electrolytes

Electrolytes are more than just a buzzword on your favorite sports drink; they are vital minerals that carry an electric charge and are pivotal to the body's fluid balance, nerve function, and muscle contractions. This chapter will unveil the intricate dance of electrolytes within your body, exploring how they maintain the delicate balance necessary for optimal physiological functioning.

Electrolytes such as sodium, potassium, calcium, magnesium, chloride, and bicarbonate play pivotal roles:

- **Fluid Balance:** They help regulate body fluids across various compartments, ensuring that hydration levels within cells and blood are appropriate.

- **Nerve Impulses:** Electrolytes are critical for the transmission of electrical signals in the body that control nerve impulses and muscle contractions.

- **Muscle Function:** Essential for muscle function, electrolytes facilitate muscle contractions and help prevent cramps.

This chapter will navigate through the essential electrolytes, delving into their specific functions, the normal levels necessary for health, and the mechanisms that keep them in check. From the muscles of an athlete sprinting to the finish line to the critical balance maintained in a patient with chronic kidney disease, electrolytes influence health and performance in profound ways.

2.1 Understanding Electrolytes

Electrolytes are minerals in your body that have an electric charge. They are in your blood, urine, tissues, and other body fluids. Electrolytes are important because they help:

- Balance the amount of water in your body
- Balance your body's acid/base (pH) level
- Move nutrients into your cells
- Move wastes out of your cells
- Make sure that your nerves, muscles, the heart, and the brain work the way they should

Major Electrolytes and Their Roles

Sodium (Na+):

- **Normal Blood Levels: 135-145 mEq/L**
- **Roles:** Sodium is crucial for maintaining fluid balance, nerve signal transmission, and muscle contraction. It helps with osmotic pressure regulation and acid-base balance which are essential for cell function.

Potassium (K+):

- **Normal Blood Levels: 3.5-5.0 mEq/L**
- **Roles:** Potassium is vital for proper cell function, including regulating heartbeat and muscle function, and conducting nerve signals. An imbalance can have serious cardiovascular and neuromuscular consequences.

Calcium (Ca2+):

- **Normal Blood Levels: 8.5-10.2 mg/dL**
- **Roles:** Beyond its well-known role in bone structure, calcium is crucial for blood clotting, nerve transmission, muscle contraction, and regulating enzyme activity.

Magnesium (Mg2+):

- **Normal Blood Levels: 1.7-2.2 mg/dL**
- **Roles:** Magnesium supports over 300 biochemical reactions in the body, including energy creation, protein formation, gene maintenance, muscle movements, and nervous system regulation.

Chloride (Cl-):

- **Normal Blood Levels: 98-106 mEq/L**
- **Roles:** Chloride helps maintain fluid balance and is an essential part of digestive stomach acids.

Bicarbonate (HCO3-):

- **Normal Blood Levels: 22-29 mEq/L**
- **Roles:** Bicarbonate regulates heart function, assists in transporting oxygen, and helps balance pH levels in the body by neutralizing acids.

Chart: Electrolyte Functions and Normal Ranges

Electrolyte	Normal Range	Primary Functions
Sodium	135-145 mEq/L	Fluid balance, nerve transmission, muscle contraction

Potassium	3.5-5.0 mEq/L	Cell function, heart stability, nerve transmission
Calcium	8.5-10.2 mg/dL	Bone health, blood clotting, muscle contraction, nerve function
Magnesium	1.7-2.2 mg/dL	Enzyme activity, nerve transmission, muscle movement
Chloride	98-106 mEq/L	Fluid balance, stomach acid production
Bicarbonate	22-29 mEq/L	pH balance, respiratory function

Understanding these electrolytes and their optimal levels is crucial for diagnosing and treating various conditions and for overall health monitoring. In clinical practice, maintaining electrolyte balance often means the difference between health and disease, making their study essential for any healthcare professional.

2.2 Major Electrolytes and Their Roles

Electrolytes are not only fundamental to maintaining fluid balance but also to various physiological processes that ensure the body operates seamlessly. Each electrolyte interacts with others and with different body systems, creating a complex network that is vital for health and well-being.

Deeper Dive into Physiological Functions and Interactions:

Sodium (Na+): Sodium is primarily responsible for controlling and regulating the volume of body fluids, an essential factor in blood pressure management. It works closely with potassium to maintain cellular function and nerve transmission. High or low levels of sodium, conditions known as hypernatremia and hyponatremia, respectively, can lead to cognitive impairment, seizures, and fluid imbalance.

Potassium (K+): Potassium is critical for muscle function, particularly in the heart where it regulates heartbeat. It works in concert with sodium to facilitate electrical gradients necessary for nerve signaling and muscle contractions. Imbalances such as hypokalemia (low potassium) can cause muscle weakness and arrhythmias, while hyperkalemia (high potassium) can lead to fatal cardiac problems.

Calcium (Ca2+): Beyond its role in bone health, calcium is crucial in muscle contractions and neurotransmitter release. It interacts with magnesium, which can compete with calcium for absorption in the body. Calcium's precise regulation is vital for ensuring that muscles can contract and relax effectively and for proper cardiac function. Hypercalcemia or hypocalcemia can lead to muscle spasms, memory loss, and arrhythmias.

Magnesium (Mg2+): Magnesium supports the function of calcium as well as potassium. It is essential for ATP production, the energy currency of the cell, and acts as a natural calcium blocker to help muscle cells relax. Low magnesium levels can exacerbate conditions like hypertension and diabetes, and lead to severe muscular and neurological symptoms.

Chloride (Cl-): Chloride, often paired with sodium, helps maintain osmotic pressure and plays a pivotal role in the body's acid-base balance. It is essential for producing stomach acid (HCl), crucial for digestion and controlling the growth of bacteria. Chloride imbalances typically accompany sodium imbalances, leading to similar symptoms such as fluid retention or loss, hypertension, and alkalosis or acidosis.

Bicarbonate (HCO3-): Bicarbonate serves as a buffer to maintain pH balance in the blood, neutralizing excess acids. It works closely with chloride and sodium to regulate acid-base balance, ensuring that metabolic processes proceed smoothly. Disturbances in bicarbonate levels can indicate kidney disease or metabolic conditions.

Clinical Significance and Examples:

- **Hypokalemia in an athlete:** Consider a long-distance runner who collapses due to severe muscle weakness and cramping. This scenario might stem from hypokalemia caused by excessive sweating and inadequate potassium intake. Immediate potassium supplementation can be crucial for recovery.

- **Hypernatremia in elderly patients:** Elderly individuals often have diminished thirst perception and could inadvertently suffer from hypernatremia, leading to neurological impairments and dehydration. Managing their fluid and sodium intake can prevent severe complications.

Understanding how these electrolytes interact and their impact on the body is essential for healthcare providers to manage conditions that stem from or result in electrolyte imbalances. Each scenario highlights the need for careful monitoring and management of electrolyte levels in different clinical situations, demonstrating the critical role they play in maintaining health and managing disease.

2.3 Electrolyte Homeostasis

Electrolyte homeostasis refers to the body's ability to maintain stable levels of electrolytes in the blood and other body fluids, despite varying dietary intake, metabolic activities, and environmental conditions. This delicate balance is crucial for proper cell function, nerve signaling, muscle contractions, and overall physiological stability. The body employs several mechanisms to achieve this balance, involving the kidneys, gastrointestinal (GI) tract, and hormonal systems.

Mechanisms of Electrolyte Regulation:

1. Renal Regulation: The kidneys play a central role in maintaining electrolyte balance by filtering blood, reabsorbing necessary electrolytes, and excreting excess amounts through urine. For example, when blood sodium levels are low, the kidneys reduce sodium excretion and reabsorb more sodium back into the bloodstream. Conversely, if blood potassium levels are high, the kidneys increase potassium excretion to prevent hyperkalemia. This finely tuned system ensures that electrolyte levels remain within narrow physiological ranges.

2. Gastrointestinal (GI) Regulation: The GI tract also contributes to electrolyte homeostasis by absorbing electrolytes from ingested food and fluids. Electrolytes like sodium, potassium, and chloride are absorbed in the intestines, and any imbalances can lead to disturbances in overall electrolyte levels. For instance, prolonged diarrhea or vomiting can result in significant losses of sodium, potassium, and chloride, leading to conditions like hypokalemia or hyponatremia.

3. Hormonal Influences: Hormones play a significant role in regulating electrolyte levels:

- **Aldosterone:** Secreted by the adrenal glands, aldosterone increases sodium reabsorption and potassium excretion in the kidneys. This hormone is particularly crucial during times of low blood pressure or low sodium levels, helping to retain sodium and water, thereby increasing blood volume and pressure.

- **Antidiuretic Hormone (ADH):** Produced by the pituitary gland, ADH helps the kidneys reabsorb water, which indirectly influences sodium concentration in the blood. It plays a key role in preventing dehydration and maintaining fluid balance.

- **Parathyroid Hormone (PTH):** Released by the parathyroid glands, PTH regulates calcium levels in the blood by increasing calcium reabsorption in the kidneys, releasing calcium from bones, and enhancing calcium absorption in the intestines. This hormone is vital in preventing hypocalcemia.

Disruptions in Electrolyte Homeostasis:

Several factors can disrupt electrolyte balance, leading to conditions with serious health implications:

- **Hypokalemia:** A condition characterized by low potassium levels, often caused by excessive loss through vomiting, diarrhea, or the use of diuretics. Symptoms include muscle weakness, cramps, arrhythmias, and fatigue. Hypokalemia can be life-threatening if severe, as it impacts cardiac function.

- **Hypercalcemia:** Elevated calcium levels in the blood can result from hyperparathyroidism, malignancy, or excessive intake of calcium or vitamin D supplements. Symptoms include nausea, vomiting, constipation, confusion, and in severe cases, cardiac arrhythmias and coma.

- **Hyponatremia:** A condition where sodium levels in the blood are abnormally low, often due to excessive fluid intake, heart failure, or certain medications. Symptoms range from headaches and confusion to seizures and coma.

Maintaining electrolyte homeostasis is a dynamic process that requires the coordinated effort of several organs and hormonal systems. Disruptions in this balance can lead to a variety of medical conditions, highlighting the importance of understanding the underlying mechanisms. Effective management of these conditions requires timely recognition and appropriate interventions to restore and maintain the delicate equilibrium of electrolytes in the body.

2.4 Clinical Implications of Imbalances

Electrolyte imbalances can have profound clinical consequences, affecting nearly every system in the body. These imbalances often present with a wide range of symptoms, some of which can be subtle, while others may be life-threatening. Proper diagnosis and treatment are crucial for restoring balance and preventing serious complications.

Common Electrolyte Imbalances and Their Clinical Impact:

1. Hyponatremia:

- **Symptoms:** Hyponatremia, or low sodium levels, often presents with symptoms such as headaches, nausea, vomiting, confusion, seizures, and in severe cases, coma. These symptoms arise from the brain swelling due to water shifting into brain cells in response to low sodium concentrations in the blood.

- **Diagnostic Criteria:** Hyponatremia is typically diagnosed when serum sodium levels fall below 135 mEq/L. It is important to assess the patient's fluid status (hypovolemic, euvolemic, or hypervolemic) to determine the underlying cause.

- **Treatment:** Treatment depends on the severity and underlying cause of the hyponatremia. Mild cases may be managed with fluid restriction, while severe cases often require intravenous saline administration. Rapid correction is avoided to prevent osmotic demyelination syndrome, a serious neurological condition.

2. Hyperkalemia:

- **Symptoms:** Hyperkalemia, or elevated potassium levels, can lead to muscle weakness, fatigue, palpitations, and potentially fatal cardiac arrhythmias. The heart is particularly sensitive to potassium levels, and high potassium can cause life-threatening arrhythmias.

- **Diagnostic Criteria:** Hyperkalemia is diagnosed when serum potassium levels exceed 5.0 mEq/L. An electrocardiogram (ECG) often shows characteristic changes, such as peaked T waves, which can help in early diagnosis.

- **Treatment:** Immediate treatment is required for hyperkalemia, particularly if ECG changes are present. Treatments may include administration of calcium gluconate to stabilize the heart, insulin with glucose to drive potassium into cells, and sodium polystyrene sulfonate or dialysis to remove excess potassium from the body.

3. Hypocalcemia:

- **Symptoms:** Hypocalcemia, or low calcium levels, can cause muscle cramps, tetany (involuntary muscle contractions), numbness, tingling, and in severe cases, seizures or cardiac arrhythmias. Chvostek's and Trousseau's signs are clinical indicators of hypocalcemia.

- **Diagnostic Criteria:** Hypocalcemia is diagnosed when serum calcium levels fall below 8.5 mg/dL. Ionized calcium, the active form of calcium in the blood, is often measured to confirm the diagnosis.

- **Treatment:** Treatment typically involves calcium supplementation, either orally for mild cases or intravenously for severe cases. Vitamin D is often administered to enhance calcium absorption from the gastrointestinal tract.

Case Studies:

Case 1: Severe Hyponatremia in an Elderly Patient An 80-year-old woman presents with confusion, lethargy, and a history of increased water intake due to perceived dehydration. Lab results reveal a sodium level of 120 mEq/L, indicating severe hyponatremia. The patient is diagnosed with euvolemic hyponatremia, likely due to syndrome of inappropriate antidiuretic hormone secretion (SIADH). Treatment includes fluid restriction and slow administration of hypertonic saline to avoid rapid shifts in sodium levels.

Case 2: Hyperkalemia in a Patient with Chronic Kidney Disease A 55-year-old man with a history of chronic kidney disease presents with weakness and palpitations. His potassium level is 6.5 mEq/L, and his ECG shows peaked T waves. Immediate treatment includes intravenous calcium gluconate to protect the heart, insulin with glucose to shift potassium into cells, and a review of his medications to identify any contributing factors, such as ACE inhibitors or potassium-sparing diuretics.

Case 3: Hypocalcemia in a Post-Thyroidectomy Patient A 45-year-old woman who recently underwent thyroid surgery presents with tingling in her hands and feet and facial muscle twitching. Her serum calcium level is 7.8 mg/dL, indicating hypocalcemia likely due to accidental removal or damage to the parathyroid glands during surgery. Treatment includes intravenous calcium gluconate and oral calcium with vitamin D to restore and maintain calcium levels.

These cases illustrate how electrolyte imbalances manifest clinically, the importance of timely diagnosis, and the tailored treatments required to manage these potentially life-threatening conditions. Understanding these imbalances and their management is crucial for healthcare providers in delivering effective patient care.

2.5 Case Studies

Case Study 1: Hyperkalemia in a Patient with Renal Failure

A 60-year-old male with a history of chronic kidney disease presented to the emergency department with complaints of severe fatigue, muscle weakness, and irregular heartbeats. On examination, his heart rate was irregular, and he appeared lethargic. An ECG showed peaked T waves, a classic sign of hyperkalemia.

Diagnostic Process: Blood tests revealed a potassium level of 7.2 mEq/L, confirming severe hyperkalemia. The patient's renal function was significantly impaired, with a glomerular filtration rate (GFR) indicating advanced kidney failure, which was the primary cause of his electrolyte imbalance.

Treatment Strategy: The treatment focused on stabilizing the patient's cardiac condition and lowering potassium levels. Intravenous calcium gluconate was administered to protect the heart, followed by insulin with glucose to drive potassium into cells temporarily. The patient was also given a cation-exchange resin to bind potassium in the intestines and was prepared for emergency dialysis to remove the excess potassium.

Outcome: The patient's potassium levels normalized following dialysis, and his symptoms improved. The ECG changes resolved, and his cardiac rhythm stabilized. This case highlights the critical role of the kidneys in maintaining electrolyte balance and the importance of prompt intervention in hyperkalemia to prevent life-threatening arrhythmias.

Learning Points:

- Hyperkalemia is a medical emergency, particularly in patients with compromised kidney function.
- ECG changes, like peaked T waves, can provide early indications of dangerous electrolyte imbalances.
- A multidisciplinary approach, including cardioprotective measures and renal replacement therapies, is essential for managing severe hyperkalemia.

Case Study 2: Hyponatremia in a Post-Surgical Patient

A 70-year-old female was admitted to the hospital following hip replacement surgery. Three days post-operatively, she became increasingly confused, lethargic, and complained of headaches. Her medical history included hypertension, for which she was taking a diuretic.

Diagnostic Process: Blood tests revealed a sodium level of 122 mEq/L, indicating moderate hyponatremia. Further investigation suggested that the use of diuretics, combined with post-operative fluid administration, contributed to the sodium imbalance.

Treatment Strategy: The patient was treated with careful fluid restriction and gradual correction of her sodium levels using isotonic saline. The diuretic was temporarily discontinued, and her electrolytes were closely monitored.

Outcome: The patient's sodium levels slowly improved, and her neurological symptoms resolved without complications. She was discharged with instructions to monitor her fluid intake and adjust her medications as needed.

Learning Points:

- Hyponatremia can develop in hospitalized patients due to medications and fluid management practices.
- Gradual correction of sodium is crucial to avoid complications like osmotic demyelination syndrome.
- Ongoing monitoring of electrolytes is essential in patients with complex medical histories or those receiving diuretics.

These case studies reinforce the importance of recognizing electrolyte imbalances early and implementing appropriate treatment strategies to prevent severe complications. They also illustrate how foundational knowledge of electrolyte physiology directly impacts patient outcomes in clinical practice.

Chapter 3: Acid-Base Balance Explained

3.0 Introduction to Acid-Base Balance

Maintaining the right acid-base balance is crucial for the body's survival. Even a slight deviation in the pH of the blood can disrupt cellular functions and lead to serious health consequences. pH, a measure of how acidic or alkaline a substance is, plays a central role in nearly every biological process. From enzyme activity to cellular metabolism, the body's pH must remain within a narrow range for these processes to function properly.

The human body constantly produces acids as byproducts of metabolism, which must be effectively neutralized or eliminated to maintain this delicate balance. The pH of blood is tightly regulated between 7.35 and 7.45, and deviations from this range can impair enzyme function, alter the structure of proteins, and disrupt the normal operation of cells and organs.

This chapter will explore the mechanisms that maintain acid-base balance, starting with the basics of pH and its importance. We'll then delve into how acids are produced and eliminated, focusing on the respiratory and renal systems' roles in this process. Additionally, we'll examine the body's buffer systems, which act as the first line of defense against pH changes. Finally, the chapter will discuss common acid-base imbalances, such as acidosis and alkalosis, and how they are recognized and managed in clinical practice.

Understanding acid-base balance is essential for anyone in healthcare, as it underpins many physiological functions and is a key consideration in patient care. This knowledge equips healthcare professionals to identify and correct imbalances, ensuring that patients maintain the optimal pH necessary for health and recovery.

3.1 Basics of pH and Its Importance

pH is a scale used to measure how acidic or alkaline a substance is, ranging from 0 to 14. A pH of 7 is neutral, while values below 7 indicate acidity and values above 7 indicate alkalinity. In the human body, pH is a crucial parameter, especially in blood, where it must be tightly regulated between 7.35 and 7.45. This slightly alkaline environment is essential for normal cellular functions and overall homeostasis.

Measuring pH: pH is measured using a logarithmic scale, which means each whole number on the scale represents a tenfold difference in hydrogen ion concentration. For example, a pH of 6 is ten times more acidic than a pH of 7. Blood pH can be measured using arterial blood gas (ABG) analysis, a common diagnostic test that provides valuable information about the body's acid-base status and respiratory function.

Normal pH Range and Its Significance: The normal pH range for human blood is 7.35 to 7.45. Deviations from this range can have significant consequences. A blood pH below 7.35 is considered acidotic, and a pH above 7.45 is considered alkalotic. Both conditions can impair cellular functions, disrupt enzymatic activities, and lead to serious health problems. For example:

- **Acidosis** can depress the central nervous system, leading to confusion, lethargy, and, in severe cases, coma.

- **Alkalosis** can cause overexcitability of the nervous system, resulting in muscle twitching, spasms, and, if left untreated, seizures.

Role of pH in Physiological Processes: pH affects several critical physiological processes:

- **Nutrient Absorption:** The acidic environment in the stomach (pH ~2) is essential for breaking down food and absorbing nutrients, particularly proteins and minerals like calcium and iron.

- **Muscle Function:** Muscle cells rely on a stable pH to function properly. During intense exercise, lactic acid builds up, temporarily lowering pH and causing muscle fatigue. The body works to buffer and remove this acid to restore normal pH and muscle function.

- **Nerve Signaling:** Nerve cells are highly sensitive to pH changes. Acidosis or alkalosis can alter the excitability of neurons, affecting how they transmit signals. This can lead to symptoms ranging from headaches and dizziness to more severe neurological impairments.

Maintaining a stable pH is vital for these and other physiological processes. Disruptions in pH balance can lead to a cascade of adverse effects, making it imperative for healthcare providers to monitor and manage acid-base levels carefully. Understanding the basics of pH and its importance is the foundation for diagnosing and treating acid-base disorders, ensuring that patients maintain optimal physiological function.

3.2 Acid Production and Elimination

The human body constantly produces acids as a natural part of metabolism. These acids must be efficiently managed to maintain the delicate acid-base balance critical for health. Understanding the sources of acid production and the mechanisms of their elimination is essential for grasping how the body controls its pH.

Sources of Acid in the Body:

1. **Metabolic Byproducts:** The primary source of acid in the body comes from metabolic processes, especially the production of carbon dioxide (CO_2). CO_2, a byproduct of cellular respiration, combines with water in the blood to form carbonic acid (H_2CO_3). This weak acid can dissociate into hydrogen ions (H^+) and bicarbonate (HCO_3^-), contributing to the body's acid load.

2. **Lactic Acid:** During anaerobic metabolism, which occurs when oxygen levels are low, muscles produce lactic acid. This often happens during intense exercise, leading to a temporary decrease in pH, which the body must buffer and eliminate to restore balance.

3. **Ketone Bodies:** In conditions such as diabetes mellitus, where glucose metabolism is impaired, the body may resort to breaking down fats for energy. This process produces ketone bodies, which are acidic and can lead to ketoacidosis if they accumulate in the bloodstream.

4. **Dietary Acids:** Foods and beverages, particularly those high in protein or processed with acids, can also contribute to the body's acid load. However, the body has mechanisms to neutralize these dietary acids effectively.

Elimination and Neutralization of Acids:

The body has three primary pathways to eliminate or neutralize acids: respiratory, renal, and chemical buffer systems.

1. **Respiratory Pathway:**

    - **Role in Acid Elimination:** The lungs play a crucial role in eliminating carbon dioxide, which indirectly helps manage acid levels. When CO_2 levels in the blood rise, the brain stimulates an increase in respiratory rate and depth, enhancing CO_2 exhalation and reducing acidity.

    - **Example:** In conditions like chronic obstructive pulmonary disease (COPD), impaired respiratory function can lead to CO_2 retention and respiratory acidosis, where the blood becomes too acidic due to insufficient CO_2 removal.

    - **Renal Pathway:**

    - **Role in Acid Excretion:** The kidneys are vital for excreting non-volatile acids (acids that cannot be exhaled) and reabsorbing bicarbonate, which acts as a buffer. The kidneys secrete hydrogen ions into the urine and generate new bicarbonate to neutralize excess acid.

    - **Example:** In metabolic acidosis, such as in renal failure, the kidneys cannot effectively excrete acid or reabsorb bicarbonate, leading to a dangerous drop in blood pH.

    - **Chemical Buffer Systems:**

    - **Bicarbonate Buffer System:** The bicarbonate buffer system is the most important extracellular buffer. It neutralizes excess hydrogen ions by forming carbonic acid, which can then be converted to CO_2, and water for exhalation or excretion.

- **Other Buffers:** Proteins, hemoglobin, and phosphate also act as buffers, neutralizing acids in the blood and within cells to prevent sudden pH changes.

Conditions Affecting Acid Production and Elimination:

1. **Respiratory Disorders:** Conditions like asthma, pneumonia, and COPD can impair the lungs' ability to remove CO_2, leading to respiratory acidosis. Conversely, hyperventilation, often caused by anxiety or pain, can lead to excessive CO_2 removal, resulting in respiratory alkalosis.

2. **Metabolic Disorders:** Diabetic ketoacidosis (DKA) is a prime example of metabolic acidosis, where the overproduction of ketones overwhelms the body's buffering capacity. Similarly, lactic acidosis can occur in shock or severe hypoxia, where anaerobic metabolism predominates.

3. **Renal Impairment:** Chronic kidney disease (CKD) hampers the kidneys' ability to excrete acids and reabsorb bicarbonate, leading to a buildup of acid in the blood (metabolic acidosis). This condition can have widespread effects, including bone demineralization and muscle wasting.

Effective management of acid production and elimination is crucial for maintaining pH within the narrow range required for life. Disruptions in these processes, whether from respiratory, metabolic, or renal disorders, can lead to significant health issues, making it essential for healthcare providers to understand and address these mechanisms in clinical practice.

3.3 Buffer Systems

Buffers are chemical systems in the body that stabilize pH by neutralizing excess acids or bases, preventing drastic changes in pH levels that could disrupt normal physiological functions. These buffers are critical for maintaining the body's pH within the narrow range necessary for enzyme activity, cellular metabolism, and overall homeostasis.

Importance of Buffers in pH Balance:

Buffers work by absorbing or releasing hydrogen ions (H^+) in response to pH fluctuations, thus maintaining a stable pH. Without these buffering systems, even minor metabolic activities or dietary changes could cause severe acid-base imbalances, leading to potential life-threatening conditions. Buffers act as the first line of defense against pH changes, working in tandem with respiratory and renal systems to ensure long-term pH stability.

Major Buffer Systems in the Body:

1. Bicarbonate Buffer System:

- **Mechanism:** The bicarbonate buffer system is the most important extracellular buffer system. It involves a dynamic equilibrium between carbonic acid (H_2CO_3) and bicarbonate (HCO_3^-) in the blood. When hydrogen ions are added to the system, they combine with bicarbonate to form carbonic acid, which can then be converted to carbon dioxide (CO_2) and water (H_2O) and exhaled by the lungs. Conversely, if the pH rises and becomes too alkaline, carbonic acid can dissociate into H^+ and HCO_3^-, thus lowering the pH.

- **Significance:** This buffer system is crucial because it can quickly respond to pH changes due to its presence in the bloodstream and its interaction with both the respiratory and renal systems. For example, during intense exercise, the body produces lactic acid, which increases H^+ concentration. The bicarbonate system rapidly buffers these excess H^+ ions, preventing a dangerous drop in blood pH.

2. **Phosphate Buffer System:**

    - **Mechanism:** The phosphate buffer system operates mainly within cells and in the urine. It consists of dihydrogen phosphate ($H_2PO_4^-$), which acts as a weak acid, and hydrogen phosphate (HPO_4^{2-}), which acts as a weak base. This system buffers acids by converting HPO_4^{2-} into $H_2PO_4^-$ when H^+ levels rise, thus reducing acidity. In the reverse scenario, $H_2PO_4^-$ can dissociate to release H^+ and HPO_4^{2-}, increasing the pH.

    - **Significance:** The phosphate buffer system is particularly important in the renal tubules, where it helps to maintain pH balance during the excretion of hydrogen ions in urine. It also plays a significant role within cells, where it buffers metabolic acids produced during energy production.

3. **Protein Buffer System:**

    - **Mechanism:** Proteins, especially hemoglobin in red blood cells, act as buffers due to their ability to bind or release

H^+ ions. Amino acids in proteins contain functional groups that can accept or donate H^+, thus buffering changes in pH. Hemoglobin, for example, binds to H^+ ions released from carbonic acid, preventing a decrease in blood pH as CO_2 is transported from tissues to the lungs.

- **Significance:** The protein buffer system is the most abundant buffer system in the body, primarily active within cells and blood plasma. Hemoglobin's role in buffering the blood during CO_2 transport is a prime example of how protein buffers maintain pH balance.

Other Buffer Systems:

- **Ammonia Buffer System:** In the kidneys, ammonia (NH_3) acts as a buffer by reacting with H^+ ions to form ammonium (NH_4^+), which is then excreted in urine. This system is especially important in chronic acidosis, where it helps to remove excess H^+ from the body.

Buffers are essential for maintaining the body's pH within its narrow, optimal range. The bicarbonate, phosphate, and protein buffer systems each play unique roles in different parts of the body, ensuring that pH balance is achieved and maintained despite the constant production of acids and bases. Understanding these systems is crucial for recognizing how the body defends against pH imbalances and for managing conditions that disrupt this delicate equilibrium.

3.4 Respiratory and Renal Contributions

The respiratory and renal systems are the two primary mechanisms the body uses to maintain acid-base balance, each playing a crucial role in regulating pH. While buffers provide an immediate response to pH changes, the respiratory and renal systems offer more sustained and adjustable mechanisms to manage long-term acid-base balance.

Respiratory Regulation of Acid-Base Balance:

The respiratory system helps regulate acid-base balance by controlling the levels of carbon dioxide (CO_2) in the blood, a key component in the formation of carbonic acid (H_2CO_3). CO_2 is a byproduct of cellular respiration and is transported in the blood to the lungs, where it is exhaled.

- **Mechanism:** CO_2 combines with water in the blood to form carbonic acid, which then dissociates into hydrogen ions (H^+) and bicarbonate ions (HCO_3^-). The concentration of CO_2 directly influences blood pH. An increase in CO_2 levels leads to the formation of more H^+ ions, lowering pH and causing acidosis. Conversely, a decrease in CO_2 levels reduces H^+ ion concentration, raising pH and causing alkalosis.

- **Compensation for Imbalances:** The respiratory system can quickly adjust to pH changes by altering the rate and depth of breathing:
    - **Hyperventilation:** In response to metabolic acidosis (e.g., diabetic ketoacidosis), the body increases the respiratory rate to expel more CO_2, reducing the acid load and helping to raise blood pH.

- **Hypoventilation:** In metabolic alkalosis, where the blood is too alkaline, the body may reduce the breathing rate to retain CO_2, which increases H^+ concentration and lowers pH back toward normal.

- **Example:** In respiratory acidosis, conditions such as chronic obstructive pulmonary disease (COPD) cause CO_2 retention, leading to increased H^+ concentration and decreased pH. The body compensates by increasing the breathing rate to expel excess CO_2 and correct the pH imbalance.

Renal Regulation of Acid-Base Balance:

The kidneys are essential for maintaining acid-base balance through their ability to excrete hydrogen ions and reabsorb bicarbonate, a crucial buffer in the blood.

- **Mechanism:** The kidneys manage pH by:

  - **Excreting H^+ ions:** The kidneys secrete H^+ ions into the urine, effectively removing them from the body. This process occurs in the renal tubules, where H^+ is exchanged for sodium ions.

  - **Reabsorbing Bicarbonate:** Bicarbonate ions, filtered out of the blood by the kidneys, are reabsorbed back into the bloodstream. This reabsorption is vital for buffering excess H^+ ions and maintaining a stable pH.

  - **Ammonium Production:** In cases of acidosis, the kidneys produce and excrete ammonium (NH_4^+), which also helps to remove excess H⁺ ions from the body.

- **Compensation for Imbalances:** The kidneys compensate for acid-base imbalances more slowly than the respiratory system but are more effective in making long-term adjustments:

- **Metabolic Acidosis:** In response to low pH, the kidneys increase the excretion of H⁺ ions and enhance bicarbonate reabsorption, gradually restoring pH to normal levels.

- **Metabolic Alkalosis:** When the blood is too alkaline, the kidneys may decrease bicarbonate reabsorption and reduce H⁺ excretion, allowing pH to decrease back toward the normal range.

- **Example:** In chronic kidney disease, the kidneys' ability to excrete H⁺ and reabsorb bicarbonate is impaired, leading to a build-up of acids in the blood and resulting in metabolic acidosis. Treatment often involves bicarbonate supplementation to help neutralize excess acid.

Integrated Response to Acid-Base Imbalances:

The respiratory and renal systems work together to correct acid-base imbalances. For example, in metabolic acidosis, the respiratory system may initially compensate by increasing CO_2 elimination (hyperventilation), while the kidneys contribute by excreting more H^+ and reabsorbing bicarbonate over time. Conversely, in respiratory alkalosis caused by hyperventilation (e.g., anxiety), the kidneys may respond by excreting bicarbonate and retaining H^+ to bring the pH back to normal.

Understanding the contributions of these systems to acid-base balance is crucial for diagnosing and managing disorders that disrupt this delicate equilibrium. The coordinated action of the respiratory and renal systems ensures that the body can effectively maintain pH within the narrow range necessary for optimal function.

3.5 Recognizing and Correcting Imbalances

Acid-base imbalances are categorized into four main types: respiratory acidosis, respiratory alkalosis, metabolic acidosis, and metabolic alkalosis. Each of these imbalances arises from either an excess or deficit of acids or bases in the body and can have significant clinical implications.

Common Acid-Base Imbalances:

1. **Respiratory Acidosis:**
    - **Cause:** Occurs when CO_2 is not effectively eliminated from the body, leading to increased blood acidity. Common causes include chronic obstructive pulmonary disease (COPD), severe asthma, or respiratory depression from medications.

- **Symptoms:** Include confusion, shortness of breath, lethargy, and, in severe cases, coma.
- **Diagnosis:** Arterial blood gas (ABG) analysis shows elevated CO_2 levels (hypercapnia) and a decreased pH.
- **Respiratory Alkalosis:**
- **Cause:** Results from excessive CO_2 elimination, often due to hyperventilation caused by anxiety, pain, or high altitudes.
- **Symptoms:** Dizziness, tingling in the extremities, and lightheadedness are common.
- **Diagnosis:** ABG shows low CO_2 levels (hypocapnia) and an increased pH.
- **Metabolic Acidosis:**
- **Cause:** Arises from an accumulation of acids or loss of bicarbonate, commonly seen in conditions like diabetic ketoacidosis, renal failure, or severe diarrhea.
- **Symptoms:** Include deep, rapid breathing (Kussmaul respiration), confusion, and fatigue.
- **Diagnosis:** ABG reveals low bicarbonate levels and a decreased pH.
- **Metabolic Alkalosis:**
- **Cause:** Often due to excessive loss of acids (e.g., from prolonged vomiting) or overuse of diuretics, leading to increased bicarbonate levels.
- **Symptoms:** Include muscle twitching, hand tremors, and nausea.

- **Diagnosis:** ABG shows elevated bicarbonate levels and an increased pH.

Clinical Recognition and Treatment:

- **Diagnosis:** Acid-base imbalances are typically diagnosed using ABG analysis, which measures pH, CO_2, and bicarbonate levels. Additional tests may include electrolyte panels and assessments of kidney and lung function to identify the underlying cause.

- **Treatment Approaches:**
  - **Respiratory Imbalances:** Focus on correcting the underlying respiratory condition. For respiratory acidosis, improving ventilation (e.g., via bronchodilators or mechanical ventilation) is key. In respiratory alkalosis, treating the cause of hyperventilation (e.g., anxiety management) is essential.
  - **Metabolic Imbalances:** Treatment involves addressing the root cause. In metabolic acidosis, bicarbonate supplementation may be necessary if the acidosis is severe. For metabolic alkalosis, correcting electrolyte imbalances and reducing bicarbonate intake are typical approaches.

Recognizing and treating acid-base imbalances promptly is crucial to preventing complications and ensuring patient recovery. The treatment must always be tailored to the specific type and cause of the imbalance, ensuring a targeted and effective response.

Chapter 4: Integration of Fluids, Electrolytes, and Acid-Base Balance

4.0 Introduction to Integration

Fluids, electrolytes, and acid-base balance are not isolated concepts; they are deeply interconnected systems that play a vital role in maintaining the body's homeostasis. Understanding how these elements interact is essential for effective clinical practice, as disruptions in one area often lead to imbalances in the others. For example, a patient experiencing dehydration might not only suffer from a loss of fluids but also from disturbances in electrolyte levels and acid-base balance, complicating their condition and treatment.

Grasping these interrelationships is crucial for diagnosing, managing, and treating a wide range of medical conditions. Whether dealing with an acute illness or managing chronic disease, healthcare providers must consider how fluid shifts affect electrolytes, how electrolyte imbalances influence acid-base status, and how all three impact overall patient health. The ability to integrate this knowledge can significantly improve patient outcomes, making it a cornerstone of competent medical care.

This chapter will explore these vital connections by examining common disorders related to fluids, electrolytes, and acid-base balance. You will learn about the physiological mechanisms that link these systems, the disorders that arise when they are disrupted, and the strategies for managing such conditions. Through practical scenarios, this chapter will also demonstrate how to apply this integrated understanding in real-world clinical settings, reinforcing the importance of a holistic approach to patient care.

4.1 Interconnections and Their Importance

The body's fluid levels, electrolyte concentrations, and acid-base balance are intricately connected through several physiological mechanisms. These systems work in harmony to maintain homeostasis, and any disruption in one can significantly impact the others, leading to a cascade of clinical complications.

Physiological Mechanisms Linking Fluids, Electrolytes, and Acid-Base Balance:

Fluids in the body are distributed between the intracellular and extracellular compartments, with electrolytes such as sodium, potassium, and bicarbonate playing key roles in maintaining this distribution. Sodium, for example, is the primary electrolyte in the extracellular fluid and is crucial for controlling fluid balance through osmosis. Potassium, on the other hand, predominates inside cells and is essential for maintaining cellular function and electrical stability.

The kidneys regulate both electrolyte levels and acid-base balance by filtering the blood, reabsorbing necessary ions, and excreting excess hydrogen ions or bicarbonate. Meanwhile, the respiratory system contributes by managing CO_2 levels, which influence the concentration of carbonic acid in the blood. Together, these systems ensure that the pH, electrolyte concentrations, and fluid volumes remain within narrow physiological ranges.

Impact of Changes in One System on the Others:

Disruptions in fluid levels, electrolyte concentrations, or acid-base balance can have immediate and far-reaching effects. For example, dehydration reduces the volume of extracellular fluid, which leads to a higher concentration of sodium (hypernatremia). This, in turn, can cause cells to shrink as water moves out to balance the extracellular sodium levels. As the kidneys attempt to conserve water, they may reduce urine output and alter the excretion of electrolytes, further complicating the body's acid-base status.

Another example is metabolic acidosis, where an excess of acid in the body depletes bicarbonate levels. The kidneys respond by excreting more hydrogen ions and reabsorbing bicarbonate, but if the acidosis is severe or prolonged, this can lead to a significant electrolyte imbalance, particularly in potassium. Hypokalemia or hyperkalemia can then cause dangerous cardiac arrhythmias, illustrating how closely linked these systems are.

Clinical Significance of These Interconnections:

Understanding the interplay between fluids, electrolytes, and acid-base balance is crucial in clinical practice. For instance, when treating a patient with diabetic ketoacidosis (DKA), a healthcare provider must address not only the elevated blood glucose levels but also the accompanying dehydration, electrolyte imbalances, and acidosis. Failure to recognize and manage these interconnected issues can lead to complications such as cerebral edema from rapid fluid shifts or life-threatening arrhythmias from potassium imbalances.

Effective patient care requires a comprehensive approach that considers how treatments for one issue might impact the others. Fluid replacement in dehydration must be carefully balanced to avoid exacerbating electrolyte imbalances or causing rapid shifts in acid-base status. Similarly, correcting an electrolyte disturbance like hyperkalemia must be done with an eye toward maintaining overall acid-base equilibrium.

In summary, the interconnections between fluid levels, electrolytes, and acid-base balance are fundamental to maintaining health and responding to illness. Clinicians must be aware of these relationships to effectively diagnose and treat conditions, ensuring that interventions in one area do not inadvertently cause harm in another.

4.2 Fluid and Electrolyte Disorders

Fluid and electrolyte disorders are common in clinical practice and can have significant consequences for patient health if not promptly identified and managed. These disorders often disrupt the delicate balance of the body's fluid levels, electrolyte concentrations, and acid-base status, leading to a range of complications. Here, we will explore some of the most common fluid and electrolyte disorders, their causes, symptoms, potential complications, and their impact on acid-base balance.

1. **Dehydration:**

    - **Causes:** Dehydration occurs when fluid loss exceeds fluid intake. This can result from excessive sweating, vomiting, diarrhea, fever, or inadequate fluid intake. It is particularly dangerous in vulnerable populations such as the elderly and infants.

    - **Symptoms:** Common symptoms include thirst, dry mouth, decreased urine output, dark urine, dizziness, and confusion. Severe dehydration can lead to hypotension, tachycardia, and shock.

    - **Complications:** Dehydration reduces blood volume, leading to hypovolemia and decreased perfusion to vital organs. This condition can also cause electrolyte imbalances, such as hypernatremia, as the body retains sodium to conserve water.

    - **Impact on Acid-Base Balance:** Dehydration can lead to metabolic acidosis due to decreased renal perfusion, which impairs the kidneys' ability to excrete hydrogen ions and reabsorb bicarbonate. This can result in a dangerous drop in blood pH, complicating the clinical picture.

2. **Overhydration (Water Intoxication):**

    - **Causes:** Overhydration occurs when there is an excessive intake of water without adequate excretion, often seen in patients with renal failure, those on certain medications (e.g., antipsychotics), or those consuming large amounts of water in a short period.

    - **Symptoms:** Symptoms include nausea, headache, confusion, and in severe cases, seizures and coma due to cerebral edema.

- **Complications:** Overhydration can dilute sodium levels in the blood, leading to hyponatremia. This can cause cellular swelling, particularly in the brain, resulting in increased intracranial pressure and potential herniation.

- **Impact on Acid-Base Balance:** The dilution of electrolytes can disrupt normal acid-base regulation, potentially leading to metabolic alkalosis if bicarbonate is retained or respiratory alkalosis if compensatory hyperventilation occurs.

3. Hyponatremia:

- **Causes:** Hyponatremia is a low sodium concentration in the blood, often caused by excessive fluid intake, renal failure, heart failure, liver cirrhosis, or the syndrome of inappropriate antidiuretic hormone secretion (SIADH).

- **Symptoms:** Symptoms range from mild (nausea, headache) to severe (confusion, seizures, coma) depending on the rate of sodium decline and the level of hyponatremia.

- **Complications:** Severe hyponatremia can lead to cerebral edema, increased intracranial pressure, and brain herniation, which are life-threatening conditions.

- **Impact on Acid-Base Balance:** Hyponatremia can exacerbate metabolic acidosis or alkalosis, depending on the underlying cause. For instance, in SIADH, where water retention is prominent, metabolic alkalosis may develop due to bicarbonate retention.

4. Hyperkalemia:

- **Causes:** Hyperkalemia is an elevated potassium level in the blood, often resulting from renal failure, potassium-sparing diuretics, adrenal insufficiency, or excessive potassium intake.

- **Symptoms:** Symptoms include muscle weakness, fatigue, palpitations, and in severe cases, life-threatening cardiac arrhythmias like ventricular fibrillation or asystole.

- **Complications:** Hyperkalemia can cause significant cardiac dysfunction, leading to sudden cardiac arrest if not promptly treated. It also affects neuromuscular function, leading to paralysis or respiratory failure.

- **Impact on Acid-Base Balance:** Hyperkalemia is often associated with metabolic acidosis, as the kidneys' ability to excrete potassium and hydrogen ions is impaired. The acidosis further exacerbates the hyperkalemia by shifting potassium from the intracellular to the extracellular space.

Clinical Implications: These fluid and electrolyte disorders not only disrupt normal physiological functions but also pose significant risks to acid-base balance. Effective management requires prompt recognition, appropriate diagnostic testing (e.g., serum electrolytes, blood gases), and tailored interventions to restore balance and prevent complications. For instance, treating hyperkalemia may involve the use of calcium gluconate to stabilize the heart, insulin to drive potassium back into cells, and diuretics or dialysis to remove excess potassium from the body.

Understanding the complex interplay between fluids, electrolytes, and acid-base balance is essential for providing high-quality patient care and improving clinical outcomes. Mismanagement of these disorders can lead to severe, even fatal, consequences, underscoring the need for a comprehensive approach to diagnosis and treatment.

4.4 Treatment Strategies

Effective management of fluid and electrolyte imbalances and acid-base disorders requires a strategic approach that addresses the underlying cause while stabilizing the patient's condition. Treatment strategies must be tailored to the individual, taking into account the severity of the imbalance, the patient's overall health, and any underlying conditions.

1. Fluid Replacement:

- **Indications:** Fluid replacement is a cornerstone of treatment for both dehydration and overhydration. In dehydration, the goal is to restore intravascular volume and correct electrolyte imbalances, while in overhydration, the focus is on reducing excess fluid volume.

- **Approach:** Isotonic solutions, such as normal saline or lactated Ringer's, are typically used for dehydration to expand extracellular fluid volume without altering electrolyte concentrations significantly. Hypotonic solutions may be used in cases of severe hypernatremia to gradually correct sodium levels. In overhydration, fluid restriction and diuretics (e.g., furosemide) may be employed to remove excess fluid while monitoring electrolyte status closely.

- **Considerations:** Fluid replacement must be carefully monitored to avoid complications such as rapid shifts in electrolytes or worsening of acid-base imbalances. For example, too rapid correction of hypernatremia can lead to cerebral edema, while aggressive fluid removal in overhydration can cause hypovolemia.

2. Electrolyte Supplementation:

- **Indications:** Electrolyte supplementation is necessary in conditions like hyponatremia, hyperkalemia, hypokalemia, and hypocalcemia. The aim is to restore normal electrolyte levels while avoiding overcorrection, which can lead to further complications.

- **Approach:** Sodium may be corrected with hypertonic saline in severe hyponatremia, while potassium supplementation can be administered orally or intravenously in hypokalemia. For hyperkalemia, calcium gluconate is often given to stabilize the heart, followed by agents such as insulin with glucose or sodium bicarbonate to drive potassium back into cells.

- **Considerations:** Electrolyte levels should be closely monitored throughout treatment. Rapid correction of imbalances, such as sodium in hyponatremia or potassium in hyperkalemia, can lead to serious complications, including cardiac arrhythmias or neurological damage.

3. Acid-Base Correction:

- **Indications:** Acid-base disorders, such as metabolic acidosis, metabolic alkalosis, respiratory acidosis, and respiratory alkalosis, require specific interventions to restore pH balance.

- **Approach:** Metabolic acidosis may be treated with sodium bicarbonate to buffer excess acid, while respiratory acidosis often requires improving ventilation to eliminate CO_2. In metabolic alkalosis, addressing the underlying cause, such as vomiting or diuretic use, and administering isotonic saline to restore chloride levels may be necessary. Respiratory alkalosis, often due to hyperventilation, may be managed with rebreathing techniques or treating the underlying anxiety or pain.

- **Considerations:** Acid-base correction must be carefully managed to avoid overcorrection. For instance, administering bicarbonate in metabolic acidosis without addressing the underlying cause can lead to a rebound metabolic alkalosis.

Tailored Approach: The success of these treatment strategies depends on a patient-centered approach that considers the individual's specific needs, underlying conditions, and potential risks. Regular monitoring of vital signs, laboratory values, and clinical status is crucial to guide treatment adjustments and ensure that interventions are both safe and effective. For example, a patient with heart failure and hyperkalemia will require careful management to balance fluid overload with the need to correct potassium levels without causing further cardiac stress.

In summary, managing fluid, electrolyte, and acid-base disorders requires a comprehensive, tailored approach that integrates clinical assessment, careful monitoring, and appropriate interventions to achieve optimal patient outcomes.

4.5 Simulated Patient Scenarios

Scenario 1: Dehydration and Hyponatremia in an Elderly Patient

Initial Presentation:
An 80-year-old woman presents to the emergency department with confusion, weakness, and a history of poor oral intake over the past few days. Her family reports that she has been experiencing nausea and vomiting. She appears lethargic and has dry mucous membranes, and her skin turgor is poor.

Laboratory Results:

- Serum Sodium: 125 mEq/L (normal: 135-145 mEq/L)

- Serum Potassium: 3.8 mEq/L (normal: 3.5-5.0 mEq/L)
- Blood Urea Nitrogen (BUN): 32 mg/dL (normal: 7-20 mg/dL)
- Serum Creatinine: 1.8 mg/dL (normal: 0.6-1.2 mg/dL)

Diagnosis and Management: The patient is diagnosed with dehydration and hyponatremia, likely due to fluid loss from vomiting and inadequate fluid intake. The initial step in management is to begin isotonic saline (0.9% NaCl) infusion to restore intravascular volume while monitoring sodium levels. The gradual correction of sodium is essential to avoid central pontine myelinolysis, a potential complication of rapid sodium correction. Regular monitoring of electrolytes, particularly sodium, and renal function is critical as the fluid status improves.

Rationale:
The isotonic saline is chosen to replenish both fluids and sodium gradually, addressing the patient's dehydration and hyponatremia without causing rapid shifts that could harm the patient's neurological function.

Scenario 2: Hyperkalemia in a Patient with Chronic Kidney Disease

Initial **Presentation:**
A 55-year-old man with a history of chronic kidney disease (CKD) presents with generalized weakness and palpitations. He reports missing his last two dialysis sessions. On examination, he has an irregular heartbeat and mild peripheral edema.

Laboratory Results:

- Serum Potassium: 6.7 mEq/L (normal: 3.5-5.0 mEq/L)

- Serum Creatinine: 5.2 mg/dL (normal: 0.6-1.2 mg/dL)
- Serum Bicarbonate: 18 mEq/L (normal: 22-28 mEq/L)

Diagnosis and Management: The patient is diagnosed with hyperkalemia due to missed dialysis sessions and CKD. Immediate management includes administering calcium gluconate intravenously to stabilize the cardiac membrane, followed by insulin with glucose to shift potassium into cells, and sodium bicarbonate to address the accompanying metabolic acidosis. Arrangements are made for urgent dialysis to remove the excess potassium from the body.

Rationale:
Calcium gluconate is prioritized to prevent life-threatening arrhythmias by stabilizing the heart. Insulin and glucose, along with bicarbonate, are used to temporarily reduce serum potassium levels while dialysis, the definitive treatment, is arranged.

Scenario 3: Metabolic Alkalosis in a Patient with Prolonged Vomiting

Initial Presentation:
A 45-year-old woman presents with severe weakness, muscle cramps, and lightheadedness. She has a history of prolonged vomiting due to a gastrointestinal infection. On physical examination, she appears dehydrated and has hypotension.

Laboratory Results:

- Serum Sodium: 137 mEq/L (normal: 135-145 mEq/L)
- Serum Potassium: 2.9 mEq/L (normal: 3.5-5.0 mEq/L)
- Serum Bicarbonate: 32 mEq/L (normal: 22-28 mEq/L)
- Blood pH: 7.49 (normal: 7.35-7.45)

Diagnosis and Management: The patient is diagnosed with metabolic alkalosis due to the loss of gastric acid from prolonged vomiting. Initial treatment involves administering isotonic saline with potassium chloride to correct hypokalemia and volume depletion. The electrolyte imbalance is monitored closely, and antiemetic medications are provided to control vomiting.

Rationale:

Saline and potassium chloride are selected to correct both the fluid deficit and the electrolyte imbalance. Potassium replacement is critical to prevent further complications, such as cardiac arrhythmias, and to help correct the alkalosis.

These scenarios demonstrate the importance of understanding the interconnections between fluid, electrolyte, and acid-base balance in clinical practice. Each case requires a tailored approach to ensure effective and safe patient care, illustrating the complexity and necessity of a comprehensive treatment strategy.

Chapter 5 Practical Applications

Mastering the concepts of fluids, electrolytes, and acid-base balance is not just about theoretical understanding—it's about applying this knowledge in real-world clinical scenarios to improve patient care. Healthcare professionals must be able to translate these concepts into practical decisions that can save lives and enhance recovery. Whether you're managing a patient in shock who requires fluid resuscitation or adjusting electrolytes in someone with chronic kidney disease, the ability to apply this knowledge effectively is crucial.

This chapter will guide you through the practical applications of what you've learned, demonstrating how these principles are used daily in clinical settings. We'll explore advanced monitoring techniques that help track fluid and electrolyte status, delve into emerging trends that are shaping the future of patient care, and provide resources to support your continuous learning in this ever-evolving field.

Understanding and implementing advanced concepts in fluid, electrolyte, and acid-base management can significantly impact patient outcomes. As you move forward in your practice, these skills will be invaluable, ensuring that your clinical decisions are informed, precise, and based on the latest evidence. This chapter will equip you with the tools and insights necessary to apply your knowledge with confidence, keeping you at the forefront of healthcare excellence.

5.1 Daily Applications

The management of fluids, electrolytes, and acid-base balance is an integral part of daily clinical practice, directly influencing patient outcomes across a wide range of medical conditions. Healthcare professionals routinely apply these concepts in various settings, from emergency departments to intensive care units, ensuring that patients receive precise and effective care.

Fluid Resuscitation in Emergency Care: In emergency care, fluid resuscitation is a critical intervention for patients experiencing hypovolemic shock due to trauma, hemorrhage, or severe dehydration. The goal is to rapidly restore intravascular volume, stabilize blood pressure, and improve perfusion to vital organs. Isotonic crystalloids, such as normal saline or lactated Ringer's solution, are commonly used to replace lost fluids without causing significant shifts in electrolyte balance. Careful monitoring is essential to avoid complications like fluid overload, which can lead to pulmonary edema, especially in patients with compromised cardiac function.

Management of Electrolyte Imbalances in Chronic Kidney Disease: Patients with chronic kidney disease (CKD) frequently suffer from electrolyte imbalances, such as hyperkalemia, due to the kidneys' reduced ability to excrete potassium. Managing these imbalances involves dietary modifications, medications like potassium binders, and, in severe cases, dialysis. Continuous monitoring of serum electrolytes is crucial to prevent life-threatening complications like cardiac arrhythmias. Tailoring treatment to each patient's needs helps maintain electrolyte homeostasis and prevent further progression of CKD.

Routine Monitoring of Acid-Base Status in Critically Ill Patients: In the intensive care unit (ICU), critically ill patients often require close monitoring of their acid-base status to detect and manage disorders such as metabolic acidosis or respiratory alkalosis. Arterial blood gas (ABG) analysis is routinely performed to assess pH, partial pressure of carbon dioxide ($PaCO_2$), and bicarbonate (HCO_3^-) levels. For example, in a patient with septic shock, metabolic acidosis can develop due to lactic acid accumulation from tissue hypoxia. Early detection and treatment with interventions like fluid resuscitation, vasopressors, and, if necessary, bicarbonate therapy are vital to correcting the acid-base disturbance and improving the patient's prognosis.

Importance of These Applications: The daily application of fluid, electrolyte, and acid-base management is pivotal in preventing complications, promoting recovery, and ultimately improving patient outcomes. Whether it's resuscitating a trauma patient, managing chronic electrolyte imbalances, or monitoring acid-base status in the ICU, these interventions are fundamental to maintaining physiological stability and supporting the body's healing processes. Understanding the nuances of these treatments allows healthcare providers to make informed, timely decisions that can make the difference between life and death.

In conclusion, the practical application of fluid, electrolyte, and acid-base management is not just routine; it is essential for delivering high-quality patient care. These daily practices ensure that patients receive the precise interventions they need to recover and thrive, highlighting the importance of a solid understanding of these critical concepts.

5.2 Advanced Monitoring Techniques

Advanced monitoring techniques are critical tools in the management of fluid, electrolyte, and acid-base balance, providing healthcare professionals with precise and real-time data necessary for effective patient care. These technologies are routinely used in hospitals and clinics to assess the physiological status of patients, guiding treatment decisions in complex cases.

Blood Gas Analysis: Blood gas analysis is one of the most important tools for evaluating a patient's acid-base status, oxygenation, and ventilation. Typically performed on arterial blood, this test measures key parameters such as pH, partial pressure of carbon dioxide ($PaCO_2$), partial pressure of oxygen (PaO_2), and bicarbonate (HCO_3^-). The results help clinicians determine whether a patient is experiencing acidosis or alkalosis and whether the underlying cause is respiratory or metabolic.

- **Technology:** Blood gas analyzers use sensors and electrodes to measure these parameters with high accuracy. The process involves drawing a small blood sample from the patient's artery, which is then analyzed in a matter of minutes, providing immediate feedback that is critical in acute settings, such as the emergency department or ICU.

- **Clinical Impact:** For instance, in a patient with suspected respiratory failure, blood gas analysis can confirm hypoventilation and respiratory acidosis, prompting the initiation of mechanical ventilation or other respiratory support measures. This real-time data is essential for making rapid and informed decisions that directly affect patient outcomes.

Serum Electrolyte Testing: Serum electrolyte testing is a routine but vital component of patient monitoring, providing information on the concentrations of key electrolytes like sodium, potassium, chloride, and bicarbonate in the blood. These tests are essential for diagnosing and managing conditions such as hyponatremia, hyperkalemia, and metabolic acidosis.

- **Technology:** Modern electrolyte analyzers use ion-selective electrodes to measure the concentration of specific ions in the blood. These analyzers are fast, reliable, and integrated into most laboratory systems, allowing for continuous monitoring of electrolyte levels, especially in critically ill patients.

- **Clinical Impact:** Accurate electrolyte monitoring is crucial in settings like dialysis units, where patients are at high risk of imbalances. For example, in a patient undergoing dialysis, monitoring potassium levels helps prevent hyperkalemia, a potentially life-threatening condition that can lead to cardiac arrest if not managed promptly.

Urine Analysis: Urine analysis is another key technique used to assess a patient's fluid and electrolyte balance. This includes testing for electrolyte excretion, osmolality, and the presence of abnormal substances such as proteins or glucose, which can indicate kidney dysfunction or other systemic issues.

- **Technology:** Automated urine analyzers use chemical reagents and optical sensors to detect and quantify various components in the urine. These systems provide rapid and comprehensive data that can guide the management of conditions like acute kidney injury or chronic kidney disease.

- **Clinical Impact:** For example, in a patient with suspected dehydration, urine osmolality and specific gravity can help confirm the diagnosis by showing concentrated urine with high electrolyte content. This information can guide fluid replacement strategies to restore proper hydration and electrolyte balance.

Potential Future Developments: The future of fluid, electrolyte, and acid-base monitoring is poised to advance significantly with the integration of new technologies. Wearable devices that continuously monitor vital signs and electrolyte levels are under development, offering the potential for real-time, non-invasive monitoring in both hospital and outpatient settings. Advances in point-of-care testing (POCT) are also likely to expand, providing immediate results in a wider range of clinical environments, from remote clinics to patients' homes.

- **Artificial Intelligence (AI) Integration:** AI and machine learning algorithms are being developed to analyze complex datasets from these monitoring techniques, offering predictive analytics that could anticipate changes in a patient's condition before they become clinically apparent. This could lead to earlier interventions and improved outcomes, especially in critical care settings.

In conclusion, advanced monitoring techniques are indispensable in the management of fluid, electrolyte, and acid-base disorders. These technologies provide the data needed for precise diagnosis and treatment, enabling healthcare professionals to deliver high-quality care. As these tools continue to evolve, they hold the promise of even greater impact on patient outcomes, driving forward the future of medical practice.

5.3 The Future of Fluid and Electrolyte Management

The management of fluids, electrolytes, and acid-base balance is undergoing significant advancements, driven by emerging trends in research, new pharmaceuticals, and innovative treatment methodologies. These developments are poised to enhance the precision, effectiveness, and personalization of patient care.

Emerging Trends and Innovations:

1. Personalized Medicine: Personalized medicine is revolutionizing the approach to fluid and electrolyte management. With the advent of genomic and proteomic technologies, it is becoming possible to tailor treatments based on a patient's genetic makeup. For example, genetic testing can identify individuals who are predisposed to electrolyte imbalances due to specific mutations affecting renal function or ion transport. This knowledge allows clinicians to anticipate potential issues and customize interventions, such as adjusting dosages of diuretics or electrolyte supplements, to better match the patient's unique physiological profile.

2. Advanced Pharmaceuticals: New pharmaceuticals are being developed to more effectively manage electrolyte imbalances and acid-base disorders. For instance, novel potassium binders, such as patiromer and sodium zirconium cyclosilicate, offer safer and more effective options for treating hyperkalemia without the risk of rapid shifts in potassium levels that can occur with older therapies. Additionally, advancements in drug formulations are improving the delivery and absorption of electrolytes, ensuring more consistent and reliable treatment outcomes, particularly in patients with chronic conditions like heart failure or chronic kidney disease.

3. Biotechnology and Wearable Devices: Biotechnology is playing a crucial role in the evolution of fluid and electrolyte management. Wearable devices that monitor electrolytes in real-time are on the horizon, offering continuous assessment of a patient's status without the need for frequent blood draws. These devices, integrated with advanced biosensors, could alert healthcare providers to impending imbalances, allowing for early intervention before clinical symptoms develop. For example, continuous glucose monitors (CGMs) have already transformed diabetes care, and similar technology for electrolytes could revolutionize the management of conditions like heart failure, where fluid and electrolyte balance is critical.

4. AI and Machine Learning: Artificial intelligence (AI) and machine learning are being increasingly integrated into clinical decision-making processes. These technologies analyze large datasets from patient monitoring systems to predict fluid and electrolyte imbalances before they become clinically apparent. AI-driven algorithms can suggest personalized treatment adjustments in real-time, optimizing fluid and electrolyte management based on the patient's current condition and historical data. This approach not only enhances precision but also reduces the likelihood of human error in critical care settings.

5. New Research Directions: Ongoing research is exploring the role of gut microbiota in electrolyte balance and acid-base regulation. Preliminary studies suggest that the gut microbiome might influence the body's handling of electrolytes and acid-base balance, opening new avenues for probiotic or microbiome-targeted therapies. Additionally, research into regenerative medicine is investigating the potential for repairing or replacing damaged renal tissues, which could dramatically improve outcomes for patients with chronic kidney disease and other conditions that affect fluid and electrolyte balance.

In conclusion, the future of fluid, electrolyte, and acid-base management is bright with possibilities. Advances in personalized medicine, biotechnology, and AI are set to transform how these critical aspects of health are monitored and treated, leading to more tailored, effective, and proactive patient care. As these innovations continue to develop, they will offer new tools and approaches that promise to improve outcomes and enhance the quality of life for patients across a range of clinical settings.

5.4 Continuous Learning

Staying current with the latest research and clinical practices in fluid, electrolyte, and acid-base management is essential for healthcare professionals. The medical field is constantly evolving, with new treatment methodologies, guidelines, and technologies emerging regularly. To provide the best care for patients, it's crucial to engage in ongoing education and professional development.

Healthcare professionals should regularly consult key textbooks such as "Fluids and Electrolytes Made Incredibly Easy!" and "The Washington Manual of Medical Therapeutics" for foundational knowledge and updates on clinical practices. Additionally, subscribing to professional journals like the "Journal of Clinical Nursing" and the "American Journal of Nursing" can provide insights into the latest research and evidence-based practices. These resources offer a wealth of information on the most current trends and recommendations in managing fluid and electrolyte imbalances.

Online courses and workshops are also valuable tools for continuous learning. Platforms such as Coursera, Medscape, and the American Nurses Association (ANA) offer a variety of courses tailored to different levels of expertise, from introductory content to advanced topics. These courses often include interactive elements, case studies, and practical applications that help reinforce learning.

Participation in professional networks and forums is another excellent way to stay informed and connected with peers. Engaging with communities such as the American Association of Critical-Care Nurses (AACN) or online forums like those on AllNurses.com allows healthcare professionals to share experiences, discuss challenges, and learn from others' perspectives. These interactions can provide practical insights and solutions that aren't always available in textbooks or formal education settings.

In conclusion, continuous learning is vital for maintaining and enhancing your skills in fluid, electrolyte, and acid-base management. By utilizing a variety of resources and engaging with the broader healthcare community, you can ensure that your knowledge remains current and that you're prepared to provide the highest level of care to your patients.

5.5 Review and Self-Assessment

As you conclude this book, take a moment to review the key concepts covered, from the basics of fluid and electrolyte balance to the intricacies of acid-base management. Below are a few self-assessment questions to help you evaluate your understanding:

1. What are the primary mechanisms by which the body maintains acid-base balance?

2. How do changes in sodium levels affect fluid balance in the body?

3. Describe the role of the kidneys in managing electrolyte imbalances.

Answers:

1. The respiratory system (via CO_2 elimination) and the renal system (via H^+ excretion and bicarbonate

reabsorption) are the primary mechanisms for maintaining acid-base balance.

2. Changes in sodium levels can lead to shifts in fluid balance, causing conditions such as dehydration or overhydration, and impact blood pressure and cellular function.

3. The kidneys regulate electrolytes by filtering blood, reabsorbing necessary ions, and excreting excess ions, thus maintaining homeostasis.

Use these questions to reinforce your learning and continue to seek out opportunities for growth in your professional practice.

Conclusion

Throughout this book, we've journeyed through the essential concepts of fluid and electrolyte balance, acid-base homeostasis, and their critical roles in maintaining health. We started with the fundamentals, understanding the distribution and movement of body fluids, and then explored the vital roles that electrolytes like sodium, potassium, and calcium play in physiological processes. We delved into the mechanisms of acid-base balance, learning how the body maintains pH within a narrow range, and how disruptions in this balance can lead to serious clinical conditions. Finally, we integrated these concepts, showing how they intersect in real-world clinical scenarios and discussing practical applications that can enhance patient care.

Understanding these topics is not just an academic exercise; it's a cornerstone of competent healthcare practice. Mastery of fluids, electrolytes, and acid-base balance equips you with the knowledge to make informed decisions, anticipate potential complications, and provide the highest standard of care to your patients. Whether you're a nursing student preparing for exams, a seasoned nurse refining your skills, or a healthcare professional seeking a deeper understanding, these concepts are fundamental to your practice.

Reflecting on the progression through this book, you've moved from basic principles to complex applications, building a robust framework of knowledge along the way. Each chapter was designed to build upon the last, gradually increasing in complexity while reinforcing the foundational concepts. This approach was intended to help you develop a deep and practical understanding of the material, even if the topics initially seemed challenging. Your commitment to engaging with this material reflects your dedication to excellence in healthcare, and for that, you should be proud.

Now, as you look forward, I encourage you to apply what you've learned in your clinical practice. Use this knowledge to make more accurate assessments, implement safer interventions, and engage in more meaningful conversations with your peers and patients. Mastery of fluid, electrolyte, and acid-base balance will not only improve patient outcomes but also enhance your confidence and competence as a healthcare provider. Remember, every piece of knowledge you've gained can directly translate into better care and better results for those you serve.

However, the learning doesn't stop here. The field of medicine is constantly evolving, and staying current with the latest research and clinical practices is crucial for ongoing professional development. I encourage you to continue your education through professional journals, online courses, and seminars. Join professional networks where you can discuss new findings and clinical experiences with colleagues. Engaging in continuous learning will ensure that your knowledge remains up-to-date and that you are always prepared to deliver the best possible care.

In closing, I want to leave you with a final thought: understanding complex medical topics like fluids, electrolytes, and acid-base balance is not only within your reach—it is essential to your role as a healthcare professional. You have the tools and the knowledge, and now it's time to use them. As you move forward in your career, remember that every patient encounter is an opportunity to apply what you've learned and to make a difference.

Thank you for dedicating your time and effort to mastering this material. I wish you continued success in your professional journey, and I hope that this knowledge empowers you to provide exceptional care. If you found this book helpful, I encourage you to share it with colleagues or students who might also benefit. Additionally, I welcome your feedback and invite you to visit our website for further resources and updates related to the topics covered in this book.

Here's to your success and to the many patients who will benefit from your expertise!

www.ingramcontent.com/pod-product-compliance
Lightning Source LLC
Chambersburg PA
CBHW070406230526
45471CB00006B/2683